Ketogenic Diet for Beginners

7-Day Ketosis Diet Plan with Healthy and Delicious Recipes for Ultimate Weight Loss

Nina Bookes

Ketogenic Diet for Beginners by Nina Bookes

Contents

Free Bonus

Wait! Before you read on I would love to share a free gift with you as a thank you for purchasing this book.

Are you struggling to lose weight or just want to lose a few pounds? Well you are not alone! If you have been searching for effective weight loss tips you have found the right place.

Right now you can get full FREE access to a downloadable e-book **'Learn the top 20 secrets to dieting success and keep the weight off forever'.**

This book is one of the most valuable resources when learning the top secrets to dieting success.

Download 'Learn the top 20 secrets to dieting success and keep the weight off forever' 100% FREE!

- Top 20 secrets to dieting success

- Practical advice on weight loss

- Tips to help you succeed

- Why these secrets are effective and much more!

Get FREE access via the last chapter of this book.

Introduction

I want to thank you and congratulate you for purchasing the book, *"Ketogenic Diet: Easy Guide to Ketosis and Losing Weight in a Healthy Way."*

Are you searching for a way to lose weight effectively and safely without any health compromises? This book contains information that might just help you. I won't promise you that it will be easy – everything good that has come into this world requires some sacrifice and a good deal of effort. BUT I can guarantee that if you follow the principles and strategies mentioned here, you will get results.

The Ketogenic Diet is one of the most effective and healthy way of losing weight. But it is also one of the most radical diets ever implemented. Many who have undertaken the diet found themselves quitting during the first few weeks due to the difficulty they've experienced or fear of the symptoms of ketosis.

However, these difficulties could have been alleviated or prevented with the right preparation and enough information about the diet. So in order to succeed and reap the benefits of the diet, you should have the right information to guide you through it.

This book contains the information you need to know as you embark on a ketogenic diet and steps on how to properly start. Reading this book will help you understand the premise of the diet, how it benefits you and whether you are at risk. You will also learn which steps to take and how to do them, such as counting calories and creating meal plans. Additionally, this book contains more than 25 recipes to enjoy and a 7-day challenge you can try for a start.

Here is a preview of what this book offers:

- Description and history of the keto diet

- Benefits from a keto diet

- Possible risks in a keto diet

- Step-by-step guide on how to begin the diet

- Breakfast recipes and many more!

Thanks again for purchasing this book, I hope you enjoy it!

What You Need to Know

The ketogenic diet and how it began

Basically, a ketogenic diet is a low-carb, moderate protein and high-fat diet. What makes it unique from other low-carb diets is that it requires *very low*, almost close to none, carbohydrate intake because a state of nutritional ketosis must be achieved.

Ketosis or the "fat-burning mode" is a metabolic state wherein the body uses ketone bodies— molecules produced by the liver from fatty acids— as its fuel source instead of the usual glucose found in carbohydrates. But in order to reach ketosis, the body must be deprived of its glucose stores. Since glucose is easier to metabolize and only a limited amount can be stored by the body, it is the body's first choice for energy.

On the other hand, fats from food that are broken down into fatty acids can either be used immediately by hungry cells or stored unlimitedly by fat cells. So in the case of a high-carb diet, fats are rarely used and mostly stored. To reach ketosis the typical macronutrient ratio of your calories should range from 60-75% fat, 15-30% protein and only 5-10% carbohydrate. Protein, which can also be used as energy, should be taken moderately because it can interfere with ketosis.

The history of the ketogenic diet began with fasting. For centuries, fasting was used as a means to treat various ailments, including seizures in children. However, prolonged starvation is detrimental to the body, so further studies were required. It was not until the early 1900s that a diet that mimics the effects of fasting was developed.

French physicians, Guelpa and Marie, were the first to report findings about the effects of fasting in epilepsy. Their report stated that seizures were significantly reduced during the treatment of 20 epilepsy patients. But still no further details were given.

In 1921, Dr. Russel Wilder proposed that a ketone-producing diet be implemented as treatment for their patients with epilepsy. He stressed the need to develop a diet that can produce the same effects of fasting but can be maintained for longer periods of time. Subsequently, he developed and coined the term "ketogenic diet." It remained popular for almost two decades, until it was replaced by the newly improved anticonvulsant medications during the early 1940s.

Its popularity was revived during the late 1990s by the story of Jim Abrahams' son, Charlie. Charlie's recovery from epilepsy through the ketogenic diet was televised and received national media attention. Charlie suffered from epilepsy since he was 2 years old. Medications and even a brain surgery were not able to help him. But when the ketogenic diet was implemented, it not only reduced the amount of seizures. It completely cured him of epilepsy.

The Charlie Foundation was then founded by his father who further increased the popularity of the diet as it funds research and helps disseminate information about the diet. Since then, the ketogenic diet has continued to rise in popularity. In recent years, the diet's popularity is due to its effectiveness in losing weight.

Benefits of a keto diet

Among current diet plans, ketogenic diet has one of the most radical metabolic shifts. Changing your energy source from carbs to fats will take at least a week or even up to a month—a phase which is undeniably difficult. To compensate for this period of suffering, a keto diet offers five major benefits, which are:

1. Keto diet is an effective treatment for Diabetes. Diabetes is a metabolic condition wherein blood sugar levels are abnormally high which when left untreated results to many complications such as ketoacidosis, cardiovascular disease, kidney failure, stroke, etc.

The abnormal sugar level can be due to either a lack of insulin in Type 1 Diabetes or insulin resistance in Type 2 Diabetes. Insulin is the key for the cells to use glucose in the blood, hence a lack of insulin production or a failure to respond to insulin leads to the accumulation of glucose in the blood.

The common treatment for any type of diabetes is a healthy diet, regular exercise and, for Type 1 Diabetes, insulin injections. And the best diet treatment for diabetes should be one which helps in maintaining the right blood sugar levels. People with diabetes are often on a blood sugar rollercoaster, wherein their blood sugar rises after a high-carb meal and drops significantly lower after an insulin injection.

A low-carb diet, such as the keto diet, is the key to lowering blood sugar and stabilizing it into unfluctuating levels. In addition, lowering the blood sugar levels will result to lower insulin levels. This reduces inflammatory damage to blood vessels, resulting to lower risks of cardiovascular disease related to diabetes.

2. Ketosis protects brain health. The brain can use either glucose or ketone bodies as energy source. Several studies revealed that ketone bodies may provide more energy per unit oxygen used than glucose. Ketone bodies also increase the brain's energy reserves by increasing the number of its mitochondria—a part of the cell responsible for energy production. Since deficient energy production is a common factor among neurological disorders, the increased energy reserve provided by the ketone bodies helps in preventing brain cell exhaustion and eventual death.

The ketogenic diet was originally intended as treatment for one of the most common neurological disorders—epilepsy. Though it is unclear how exactly it works, many case studies prove the efficacy of the ketogenic diet as treatment to epilepsy, especially for children. This is a commonly recommended treatment for children since it is natural and does not involve medicated drugs. More than 50% of the children who had undergone this treatment experienced positive results. Some children showed significant decrease of seizures while others were cured completely.

Due to the success of the ketogenic diet in treating epilepsy, further studies about its effect on other neurodegenerative disorders were conducted. For example, studies on Alzheimer's Disease showed that the keto diet can aid in relieving its symptoms and possibly reverse its degenerative process.

3. *A high-fat diet helps maintain a healthy cardiovascular system.* For years, it has been taught that fat contributes to heart diseases and other cardiovascular problems. It is no wonder why people would negatively react to any suggestions of increasing fat intake, since they have known that fat is always at the top of the food pyramid. Fortunately, recent studies have debunked this myth and proved that a keto diet is actually beneficial to the heart.

Fats in our bloodstream have two forms, cholesterol and triglycerides. Contrary to common belief, cholesterol is an important molecule needed by the body for many functions such as vitamin absorption, hormone build-up, and cell maintenance. Triglycerides, on the other hand, functions as energy stores. In other words, adequate amount of fats is needed by the body to function well.

HDL, or the good cholesterol, is one of the lipoproteins that transport cholesterol throughout the body. HDL is called *good* because it not only transports the cholesterol. It also collects and delivers unused cholesterol back to the liver. As a result, it clears the arteries of unwanted molecules that can contribute to clogging. A keto diet increases HDL in the bloodstream which is necessary for maintaining a healthy cardiovascular system.

The culprit for the bad reputation of fats is the LDL, commonly known as the bad cholesterol. Like the HDL, it is not just cholesterol but a transporter as well. The LDL, however, move more slowly thus have a tendency to clog the blood vessels. A keto diet reduces LDL levels and increases the size of their molecules, making them less harmful.

4. A keto diet can also aid in fighting cancer. Excess sugar consumption contributes to many known types of cancer. That is because cancer cells thrive on glucose. Hence, the more glucose you have in your bloodstream, the more you allow cancer cells to thrive and possibly grow out of control.

What happens then on a low-carb diet? As blood glucose and insulin levels drop, cancer cells are deprived of their fuel source and starved to death. This means a keto diet is not only a preventive measure against cancer, but also an alternative treatment or a complimentary treatment for those who have cancer.

5. It is an effective way to safely lose weight. Ketosis can help you lose weight in two ways: First, it burns stored fats for energy, so your total body fats decreases. Second, it helps the body regulate balanced hormones. Unbeknownst to many, the root cause of weight gain is hormonal imbalance, specifically the insulin.

Insulin is the hormone responsible for moving the glucose into the cells where it can be used as fuel. When you consume a high-carbohydrate diet, glucose in the bloodstream increases. This causes the brain to signal the pancreas to release more insulin to manage the glucose. An excessive intake of carbs leads to high levels of insulin.

When your insulin levels are abnormally high, the cells cannot use stored fats, thus, they become dependent solely on glucose for energy. In severe cases, cells become very dependent on the glucose from food rather than their stored energy.

This manifests as extreme hunger and it is the reason why people crave carbs and tend to overeat, which will eventually lead to weight gain. In addition to hunger, hormonal imbalance can also result to low energy levels. People who get easily fatigued struggle with proper exercise and settle on sedentary lifestyles.

Fortunately, the keto diet can lower both blood sugar and insulin levels. It helps your hormones stay balanced and keep you satiated, preventing you from overeating. Furthermore, energy from fats last longer throughout the day which can help you live a more active lifestyle.

Dangers in a keto diet

You may have heard how a ketogenic diet can be dangerous. The most common basis for this assumption is because ketogenic diet is originally implemented under medical supervision and used for people with certain illnesses. However, modern studies have modified the current keto diet for anyone who wants to achieve weight loss and gain health benefits.

Another possible basis for their fear is due to the life-threatening metabolic condition called ketoacidosis. There is some confusion between ketosis and ketoacidosis. Some believe that prolonged ketosis may lead to ketoacidosis, while others simply do not know the difference.

Ketosis is a normal body response due to the shift in body chemistry. Therefore, it is not, as some may believe, a dangerous health condition. On the other hand, ketoacidosis is an abnormal metabolic condition wherein the body can no longer regulate ketone production resulting to excessive ketone bodies in the bloodstream. This condition can be fatal. In addition, ketoacidosis is commonly a complication of Type 1 Diabetes. It results from irregular insulin production and not from prolonged ketosis.

However, people who require a high protein diet and people at risk of ketoacidosis and those with chronic metabolic conditions should not get into this diet or should at least be under the supervision of a physician. They include pregnant and lactating women, children, people with anorexia, people prone to kidney stones, people with metabolic disorders that inhibits normal fat metabolism, and those with pancreatic disorders or insulin insufficiency.

Steps on How to Begin a Keto Diet

Step 1: Know your body

As we have stated in the previous chapter, there are possible risks in undertaking a ketogenic diet. You have to be ruled out from the category of people who are at risk before you start. Hence, the first step is to talk to your physician.

Once you know that it is safe for you to carry on, identify your body mass index or BMI to get your ideal body mass. You will be able to categorize whether you are underweight, normal or overweight. Though the BMI does not accurately measure your body fat or muscle mass, it can serve as a baseline measurement that you can use to track your progress in losing weight. You can use an online BMI Calculator.

For example, a 25-year old female who weighs 122 pounds with a height of 5 feet and 4 inches, has a BMI of 20.94 kg/m². Her BMI is within the normal range, so her ideal calorie intake is that which maintains her weight.

The next thing you have to identify is your recommended calorie intake, since the amount of calories we need varies depending on our gender, age, height, weight and level of activity. Use an online Calorie Calculator to estimate the calorie you need per day. The calculator gives both the recommended amount for maintenance and fat loss.

Using the example above, the recommended amount for her to maintain her weight is 1,540 calories per day; and the recommended amount for her to lose 1 pound per week is 1,040 calories per day.

Keep in mind that these are only approximate values and that there are other factors that affect weight loss, such as the person's metabolic rate, the effectiveness of her endocrine system, etc. Therefore, results may vary from person to person. You can adjust your calorie intake according to the results at the end of each week. Add 5 to 10% to your calories if you lost more than what you intended and reduce if you lost less.

Step 2: Learn how to calculate calories and nutrients of a meal

To be able to comply with your recommended calorie intake, you have to calculate how much calories and macronutrients each meal contains. You can do it manually or use a software wherein you simply type in the name and amount of each ingredient to automatically get the numbers. To compute manually, you have to determine the calorie and nutrient content of each ingredient by checking the label or researching the USDA National Nutrient Database or other websites. Then get the total of their calorie and macronutrient content.

Example: Simple ribeye steak recipe

Ingredient	Calorie	Fat	Protein	Carb
1lb. ribeye steak	1243	100g	79g	0
1tsp. animal fat*	38	4g	0	0
Salt and pepper	3	0	0.1g	0.7g
Total	1284	104g	79.1g	0.7g
Per serving (3)	428	34.67g	26.37g	0.23g

* Only 1 tsp. is absorbed by the meat from the original 3 tbsps. in the recipe.

Once you know the nutrient and calorie content of your food options, you'll be able to identify which items to buy and how much of each to take.

Step 3: Reorganize and restock your kitchen

Now that you have all the information you need, it's time to take action. Throw away all the junk from your kitchen and refill it with keto-friendly foods. Junk foods include white rice, white bread, refined sugar or any food that has refined sugar, highly processed foods, etc. Besides from junk foods, you should also remove any food with high-carb content such as starchy vegetables and most fruits.

Since the diet is basically reducing your carbs and increasing your dietary fats with moderate protein intake, you should shop for fattier cuts of meat, a selection of healthy fats and oils, low-carb fruits and vegetables, and full-fat dairy products. It is best to choose foods that are closest to their natural forms.

For a healthier diet, follow these basic guidelines:

- Choose organic fruits and vegetables to avoid consuming pesticides and added chemicals.

- Choose meat from wild-caught, free-ranged and grass-fed animals to avoid consuming injected antibiotics or growth hormones and promote a more humane treatment for the animals.

- Choose plant-based milk such as almond milk, rice milk, soy milk and coconut milk.

- Choose cold-pressed vegetable oils and limit intake of oils rich in Omega-6 fatty acid such as canola oil, sunflower oil, nut oils, etc.

Day	Breakfast	Lunch	Dinner	Dessert/ Snack
Mon	Chicken Sausage and Mushroom Frittata (240 calories)	Simple Ribeye Steak (428 calories)	Hot and Cheesy Chicken Casserole (636 calories)	2 Cheddar Cheese Chips (108 calories)
Tue	Leftover Frittata (240)	Leftover Chicken Casserole (636)	Baked Herbed Salmon (353)	Keto Strawberry Ice Cream (178)
Wed	Coconut Pecan Fat Bombs (303); 2 cups almond milk (80)	Keto Capresse Salad (405)	Keto Crockpot Lamb (524)	Keto Clam Chowder (183)

Thu	Breakfast Smoothie (261)	Leftover Crockpot Lamb (524)	Shrimp Scampi with Spinach (390)	30g Macadamia nuts (215)
Fri	1 almond bun with 2 tbsps. peanut butter (454)	Moroccan Lamb Chops (519)	Oriental Chicken Dish (362)	2 large beef jerky strips (164)
Sat	Berry Coconut Smoothie (261)	Zesty Chicken Breast (649)	Grilled Short Ribs (417)	30g almonds (173)
Sun	Cinnamon Spice Waffles (542)	Leftover Grilled Short Ribs (417)	Rosemary and Thyme Crockpot Lamb (414)	1 large hard-boiled egg (78)

Replace sugar with natural low-carb sweeteners such as erythritol, stevia, xylitol, and yacon syrup.

Step 4: Learn how to cook and create a meal plan

Cooking your own meals is the key to controlling your food intake and creating a meal plan is essential in keeping a balanced diet. The following chapters will give you a few samples of recipes that you can try out for a start. Once you get used to cooking meals, eventually, you'll be able to come up with your own recipes.

When creating a meal plan, keep in mind the ideal ketogenic ratio for calories; that is, 72% fat, 23% proteins, and 5% carbs. You can get the estimated values by using a Keto Calculator, which is available online. For example, a 1500-calorie diet is equal to 122g fat, 83g protein and 19g carbs daily.

Follow this 7-day challenge for a recommended 1500 calories per day as an example:

The meals total calorie per day should be more or less than 1500 calories. Fat content should be around 115-125g, while protein ranges from 83-93g, and fat is less than 20g.

Step 5: Keep a food diary

Meal	Food and Amount	Calories	Notes
Breakfast	1 glass breakfast smoothie 1 ½ glass of water 1 small apple	261 80	Got hungry, grabbed an apple on my way to work
Lunch	1 slice of the leftover casserole 1 serving of strawberry ice cream	636 178	The ice cream satisfied my cravings for sweets

Keeping a food diary has many benefits. It tracks your calorie intake and helps you balance it throughout a week or a month. It helps you discover your food intolerances or foods that aggravate a health condition. It can also make it easier for your physician or nutritionist to help you with a health condition.

To create a food diary, simply jot down the food you ate and take note of your body's reaction or how you felt.

Example:

Also, on another table, write down any additional information such as the condition of your sleep on the previous night, or your activities and mood swings during the day. You can modify this table to include additional information. Other food logs include the nutrient content, the specific time they ate and even where they ate.

Additional tips for achieving success in keto

- If you find computing the right ratio of macronutrients an inconvenience, then just remember to keep your net carbohydrate intake below 20g per day. If the label only shows the total carb content, subtract the fiber grams from the total to get the net carbs. Choose foods and ingredients that have low-carb content.

- Test whether you are in the state of ketosis. It is important to know whether the diet is working on you. Knowing that it is will also encourage you to continue despite the difficulties of the initial process. Ketone testing kits are available in most drugstores and are usually cheap and easy to use.

- You'll need to drink plenty of water on a low carb diet because the body does not retain water the same way. Glucose from carbohydrates is stored with lots of water; so when the body is dehydrated, it turns to its stored glucose to use the water. Consequently, on a low-carb diet, you will feel incredibly thirsty especially during the first weeks of adjusting. Never ignore thirst because it is your body's signal that it needs water. Drink at least 3 liters of water per day.

- Dehydration involves more than just the lack of water. There is also a deficiency of important electrolytes such as sodium, potassium, magnesium, etc. This often leads to symptoms such as heart palpitations, headaches, cramps, etc. To prevent these deficiencies, increase the salt in your diet and take potassium and magnesium supplements.

- Aside from electrolytes, fiber is also inadequate in a low carb diet. Many of the most common sources of fiber are high-carb foods which you are now avoiding. Deficiency in fiber may lead to constipation.

So you need to increase non-starchy vegetables, flaxseed meal and psyllium seed husks in your diet. Eat leafy greens alongside your main meal or add flaxseed meal and psyllium seed husks to your baked goods.

- Be aware of the side-effects during the adjusting period of the body and try not to panic. Common symptoms include frequent thirst, constipation, decreased appetite, dizziness and flu-like symptoms. Many dieters have quit thinking that keto diet is dangerous because of the symptoms of sugar or carb withdrawal. Fortunately, these symptoms can be alleviated by drinking water, eating the right food or taking supplements. Whenever you find yourself craving for carbs or sweets, eat something you like that complies with the keto diet.

- Avoid getting hungry. Once you get hungry, it becomes harder to fight off your carb cravings and other indulgences. The solution is to eat a lot of satisfying foods that are keto-friendly. Eating foods that make you happy and satisfied is an important factor that helps you stay on any diet plan.

Breakfast Recipes

Keto Cinnamon Spice Waffles

Ingredients:

(Waffle batter)

2 large eggs

½ tsp cinnamon powder

6 tbsps. almond flour

¼ tsp. baking soda

1 tbsp. erythritol (or other natural sweetener of your choice)

½ tsp. vanilla extract

(Cream cheese filling)

2 tsps. batter

¼ tsp. cinnamon

1 tbsp. heavy cream

2 tbsps. cream cheese

1 tbsp. erythritol

¼ tsp. vanilla extract

Instructions:

1. In a mixing bowl, beat one egg with the erythritol. Add in the cinnamon and almond flour, then mix well. Make sure there are no lumps left. Then add in the other egg, vanilla extract and baking soda. Mix well until smooth.

2. Pre-heat your non-stick waffle maker. If you don't have a waffle maker then don't fret. You can use a griddle or you can also use a grill pan. You also need to preheat the griddle/grill pan on high heat but set it down to medium when you start to pour waffle mixture on it. Once it's hot enough, pour in your batter. Set aside at least 2 teaspoons of batter for the filling.

3. Meanwhile, in a small bowl, combine the cream cheese and erythritol. Then add in the leftover batter, cinnamon, vanilla extract and heavy cream. Mix well until thoroughly combined.

4. Take out your waffles and serve them with the filling. You can cut your waffles into a smaller size to make a sandwich with the filling.

Nutrition Information

Serves: 1-2

Calories: 542

Fats: 50g, Net Carbohydrates: 7g, Fiber: 6g, Protein: 22.8g

Coconut Pecan Fat Bombs

Ingredients:

½ cup shredded coconut (unsweetened)

2 cups pecans (cut into halves)

½ cup golden flaxseed meal

1 cup almond flour

½ cup coconut oil

25 drops stevia (or other natural liquid sweetener of your choice)

¼ cup *keto maple syrup* (recipe included)

Instructions:

1. Preheat oven to 350°F. Bake pecan halves for about 6 to 8 minutes. Remove from oven and let them cool for a few minutes. Then place them in a plastic bag and crush them into large pieces using a rolling pin. The size depends on you.

2. In a mixing bowl, thoroughly combine shredded coconut, flaxseed meal and almond flour. Then add in the pecan chunks and mix again. Finally, mix in all the liquid ingredients to form the dough.

3. Place the dough in an 11 x 7 baking dish. Press the dough until the top is even.

4. Place in a preheated oven at 350°F. Bake for about 20 to 25 minutes.

5. Remove from the oven and set aside to cool for a few minutes. Refrigerate for at least an hour. Then slice into 12 pieces or bars. You can serve with extra pecans for toppings.

Nutrition Information

Yields: 12 bars

Calories: 302.6 (per bar)

Fats: 30.5g, Net Carbohydrates: 2g, Fiber: 4.5g, Protein: 4.9g

Keto Maple Syrup

Ingredients:

2 tsps. maple extract

¾ cup water

1 tbsp. butter (unsalted)

2 ½ tsps. coconut oil

¼ cup erythritol (or other natural powdered sweetener of your choice)

¼ tsp. xanthan gum

½ tsp. vanilla extract

Instructions:

1. Combine coconut oil, butter and xanthan gum in a container and microwave for 40 seconds.

2. Add in erythritol and water. Mix well then add the remaining ingredients. Mix again until thoroughly combined.

3. Microwave again for 50 to 60 seconds. Let it cool before serving.

Nutrition Information

Yields: 1 cup

Serves: 4

Calories: 49 (per ¼ cup), Fats: 5.5g, Net Carbohydrates: 0, Fiber: 1g, Protein: 0

Keto Omelet with Goat Cheese

Ingredients:

3 large eggs

1 handful fresh spinach

1 oz. goat cheese (crumbled)

2 tbsps. butter

2 tbsps. heavy cream

¼ medium white onion (sliced into long strips)

1 spring onion (for garnish)

Sea salt and pepper to taste

Instructions:

1. In a medium skillet, melt butter over low heat until it begins to brown. Then sauté the onion until it caramelizes.

2. Then add the spinach and let it cook until the leaves wilt. Season with salt and pepper to taste. Remove from heat and set aside.

3. In a small mixing bowl, beat the eggs with the heavy cream and season with salt and pepper to taste. Combine thoroughly.

4. Preheat the skillet into medium-low heat. Once it's hot, gently pour in the egg mixture and let it cook.

5. Before the top completely sets, place the spinach mixture onto half of the omelet. Top it with the crumbled goat cheese. Then fold it in half. Serve immediately and garnish with chopped spring onions.

Nutrition Information

Serves: 1

Calories: 620

Fats: 56g, Net Carbohydrates: 5.5g, Fiber: 1g, Protein: 25g

Baked Chicken Sausage and Mushroom Frittata

Ingredients:

10 large eggs

2 ½ cup Bella mushrooms (sliced)

3 cups fresh spinach (roughly chopped)

3 chicken sausages (sliced horizontally)

1 ½ cup cheddar cheese

2 tsps. hot sauce

1 tbsp. ranch dressing

½ tsp. Mrs. Dash Table Blend seasoning (or other seasoning of your choice)

Sea salt and pepper to taste

Instructions:

1. Preheat oven to 400°F.

2. Preheat a cast iron skillet over medium-high heat. Once heated, cook sausage slices until crisp on one side. Then turn them over and

add the spinach and mushrooms. Leave them to cook.

3. Meanwhile, beat the eggs in a mixing bowl with the seasoning, hot sauce and ranch dressing. Mix thoroughly.

4. Stir the sausages, mushrooms and spinach, then season with salt and pepper to taste.

5. Add the shredded cheddar cheese on top. Then pour in the egg mixture. Stir well until the egg mixture reaches the bottom of the skillet.

6. Transfer the skillet to the oven and bake for 10 minutes. Then broil the top for another 3 minutes.

7. Remove from the oven and set aside to cool. Cut into 8 pizza slices and serve.

Nutrition Information

Serves: 8

Calories: 240 (per slice)

Fats: 17.75g, Net Carbohydrates: 2.2g, Fiber: 0.9g, Protein: 19.9g

Berry Coconut Breakfast Smoothie

Ingredients:

¼ cup fresh blueberries

2 cups coconut milk (unsweetened)

1 tbsp. chia seeds

3 tbsps. golden flaxseed meal

2 tbsps. MCT oil

10 drops stevia (or any natural liquid sweetener of your choice)

7 ice cubes

Instructions:

1. Using a blender, combine coconut milk, ice cubes and liquid stevia. Pulse until smooth.

2. Add in the blueberries, flaxseed meal and chia seeds. Wait for a few minutes to allow them to soak in the liquid. Then blend until thoroughly combined. Pour in a glass and serve. You can add extra blueberries for toppings.

Nutrition Information

Serves: 2

Calories: 261 (per glass)

Fats: 25g, Net Carbohydrates: 3g, Fiber: 7g, Protein: 4g

Poultry Recipes

Zesty Chicken Breast

Ingredients:

1 lb. chicken breast fillet (skinless and boneless)

1 lemon (juiced)

¾ cup olive oil

15 pcs. olives

2 oz. camembert

1 tbsp. ground rosemary

Sea salt and pepper to taste

Instructions:

1. In a mixing bowl, combine the lemon juice, rosemary, olive oil and a pinch of pepper to make the marinade. Mix well until thoroughly incorporated.

2. Chop chicken breasts into cubes and marinate for a minimum of 2 hours in the

refrigerator. Season with salt after refrigerating.

3. Preheat a non-stick skillet over medium heat. Once hot, cook the chicken with the marinade until the liquid evaporates.

4. Transfer on a plate and serve with olives and camembert on the side.

Nutrition Information

Serves: 3

Calories: 603 (per serving)

Fats: 50g, Net Carbohydrates: 1.3g, Protein: 42g

Keto Oriental Chicken Dish

Ingredients:

2 chicken thighs (with skin, deboned)

¼ cup peanuts

2 spring onions (chopped)

4 red Thai chilies (deseeded and chopped)

½ green pepper (diced)

1 tsp. ground ginger

Sea salt and pepper to taste

(Sauce ingredients)

2 tbsps. chili garlic paste

1 tbsp. soy sauce

1 tbsp. ketchup (reduced sugar)

2 tsps. Sesame oil

2 tsps. Cider vinegar

10 drops stevia (or any natural liquid sweetener of your choice)

½ tsp. maple extract

Instructions:

1. Chop chicken thighs into bite-sized pieces and season with ginger powder, salt and pepper.

2. Preheat non-stick skillet over medium-high heat. Once hot, cook chicken for about 10 minutes or until browned.

3. While cooking the chicken, combine all sauce ingredients in a small mixing bowl and mix well.

4. Once the chicken browned, stir in chopped veggies, chilies and peanuts. Cook for another 3 minutes or until the veggies are tender. Then pour in the sauce and let it boil until it thickens. Serve hot.

Nutrition Information

Serves: 3

Calories: 362 (per serving)

Fats: 27.4g, Net Carbohydrates: 3.2g, Fiber: 1.3g, Protein: 22.3g

Hot and Cheesy Chicken Casserole

Ingredients:

6 chicken thighs (small)

3 jalapenos (medium)

¼ cup hot sauce (low-carb)

¼ cup mayonnaise

12 oz. cream cheese

2 oz. mozzarella cheese (shredded)

4 oz. cheddar cheese (shredded)

Salt and pepper to taste

Instructions:

1. Preheat oven to 400°F.

2. Remove the bones from the chicken thighs and season with salt and pepper. Place them on a wire rack over a cookie sheet lined with foil. Then bake for 40 minutes.

3. Meanwhile, cook jalapenos in a pan over medium heat. If you prefer it to be less spicy,

remove the seeds before cooking. Then add in hot sauce, cream cheese and mayonnaise. Season with salt and pepper to taste. Stir well.

4. Take out the chicken from the oven and set aside to cool for a few minutes. Then remove skins and place in a single layer on a casserole dish.

5. Pour the cream cheese and jalapeno mixture over the chicken thighs and spread evenly. Top with mozzarella and cheddar cheese.

6. Bake for 12 minutes at the same temperature and broil for another 5 minutes. Let it cool for 5 minutes before slicing, then serve.

Nutrition Information

Serves: 6

Calories: 636 (per

Fats: 51g, Net Carbohydrates: 2.5g, Fiber: 0.2g, Protein: 29g

Keto Chicken Balls

Ingredients:

1 chicken breast

2 tbsps. almond flour

1 medium egg

15g grated parmesan cheese

½ tsp. baking powder

1 tbsp. water

Instructions:

1. Cook chicken breast for about 10 minutes. Then chop it into cubes.

2. Thoroughly combine all ingredients using a food processor.

3. Preheat your deep fryer. Divide mixture into 1-inch balls and drop them into the hot frying oil. Turn them frequently to avoid sticking at the bottom. Cook for about 5 minutes or until

golden brown. Serve immediately with your favorite side dish.

4. If you want to deep fry your meatballs and avoid the extra oil then you can bake your meatballs instead. Preheat your oven to medium (somewhere around 400 degrees or less – depends on the oven you're using; there are some electric ovens have lower max temperature settings).

5. Line baking sheet with parchment paper and lightly spray some oil on it so the chicken balls don't stick. Arrange the chicken balls about an inch apart on the sheet. Bake them for about 20 minutes (if you made bigger chicken balls then bake for 25 minutes or until they're done).

Nutrition Information

Serves: 2

Calories: 166 (per serving)

Fats: 9g, Net Carbohydrates: 2g, Fiber: 1g, Protein: 23g

Quick and Easy Buffalo Wings with Bleu Cheese Dip

Ingredients:

18 chicken wings

4 tbsps. butter (melted)

4 tbsps. hot sauce (choose low carb or less sugar)

(7 oz. Bleu cheese dip)

3 oz. bleu cheese (crumbled)

1 oz. cream cheese

2 oz. mayo

1 oz. sour cream

½ tbsp. lemon juice

Instructions:

1. Preheat oven at 450°F.

2. In a sturdy container, combine all ingredients for the dip and mix thoroughly using an immersion blender. Blend until you achieve desired consistency. You can also set

aside a few crumbled bleu cheese before blending them, then add it afterwards for added texture. Set aside the dip.

3. Cover a baking tray with foil and lightly grease it with oil. Place the chicken wings and bake for 20 minutes. Then flip them and bake for another 15 minutes.

4. Meanwhile, combine melted butter and hot sauce. Mix until fully combined.

5. Remove from oven and evenly coat the wings with the sauce. Place them on a plate and pour the remaining sauce over the wings. Serve with the bleu cheese dip.

Nutrition Information

Serves: 2 (9 wings each)

Calories: 1185 (per serving)

Fats: 103g, Net Carbohydrates: 2g, Protein: 60g

Beef and Lamb Recipes

Oriental Grilled Short Ribs with Sesame seeds

Ingredients:

6 short ribs (flanken cut)

2 tbsps. fish sauce

¼ cup soy sauce

2 tbsps. rice vinegar

½ tsp. sesame seeds

1 tsp. ground ginger

½ tsp. garlic (minced)

½ tsp. onion powder

¼ tsp. cardamom

½ tsp. red pepper flakes

1 tbsp. sea salt

Instructions:

1. In a mixing bowl, combine the soy sauce, fish sauce and rice vinegar to make the marinade.

2. Put short ribs in a casserole dish and pour over the marinade. Let it marinate for 1 hour.

3. In another bowl, combine all the remaining ingredients to make the spice rub. Mix well until fully incorporated.

4. Drain the marinade from the short ribs and rub the spice mixture evenly into each rib. Make sure to cover all sides.

5. Preheat the grill. Once hot, cook the ribs for about 3 to 5 minutes on each side. Then serve immediately.

Nutrition Information

Serves: 4

Calories: 417 (per serving)

Fats: 32g, Net Carbohydrates: 0.9g, Protein: 29.5g

Simple Tender Ribeye Steak

Ingredients:

2 ribeye steaks (medium)

3 tbsps. ghee or just plain butter

Kosher salt and pepper to taste

Instructions:

1. Preheat oven to 250°F.

2. Season the steaks with salt and pepper. Make sure that all sides are evenly coated. Then place them on a wire rack atop a baking sheet.

3. Place in the oven and bake for about 40 to 45 minutes. Afterwards, take them out and set aside for a few minutes to rest.

4. Meanwhile, preheat a cast iron skillet and heat the cooking fat until smoking point. Then sear all sides of the steaks for about 30 seconds. Let them rest for 2 minutes before serving. Serve warm with your favorite side dish.

Nutrition Information

Serves: 3

Calories: 428 (per serving)

Fats: 34.67g, Net Carbohydrates: 0.23g, Protein: 26.37g

Keto Moroccan Lamb Chops

Ingredients:

8 lamb loin chops

2 tbsps. ras el hanout (a Moroccan spice mix) or ground pepper and cumin

1 tsp. olive oil

Sea salt to taste

(Charmoula marinade)

3 garlic cloves (chopped)

¼ cup olive oil

2 tbsps. lemon zest

2 tbsps. lemon juice

2 tbsps. fresh mint (chopped)

½ tsp. paprika

¼ cup fresh parsley (chopped)

1 tsp. red pepper flakes

Sea salt and freshly ground pepper to taste

Instructions:

1. Coat the lamp chops with olive oil and rub with salt and spice mix.

2. Preheat grill. Once hot, cook the lamb chops for about 2 to 3 minutes on each side. Set aside for a few minutes.

3. Meanwhile, use a food processor to combine and blend all the ingredients for the charmoula. Make sure not to over blend. It should have a little texture to it.

4. Serve lamb chops drizzled with the charmoula and lemon zest.

Nutrition Information

Serves: 4

Lamb chops (2 pieces), Calories: 392, Fats: 29g, Net

Carbohydrates: 0, Protein: 31g

Charmoula (2 tbsps.), Calories 127, Fats: 14g, Net

Carbohydrates: 1.5g, Protein: 0

Ketogenic Diet for Beginners by Nina Bookes

Keto Crockpot Lamb

Ingredients:

1 lamb leg (with bone)

¼ cup fresh mint leaves (finely chopped)

6 cups green beans (trimmed)

4 cloves garlic (thinly sliced)

2 tbsps. ghee or any cooking fat of your choice

Sea salt and freshly ground black pepper to taste

Instructions:

1. Season the lamb leg with salt and pepper to taste. Make sure to evenly coat all sides.

2. Melt ghee in a large pot over medium heat. Place the lamb and fry until golden brown. Make sure to brown both sides. Then remove from heat.

3. Place the lamb in a crock-pot and sprinkle the chopped mint and sliced garlic all over it. Then add half a cup of water, cover with its lid and cook for 10 hours on low. If you want to cook faster, set on high and cook for about

6 hours. Add the green beans when you only have 2 hours left of cooking time.

Nutrition Information

Serves: 4

Calories: 524 (per serving)

Fats: 36.4g, Net Carbohydrates: 7.6g, Fiber: 4.4g, Protein: 37g

Rosemary and Thyme Crockpot Lamb

Ingredients:

2 lbs. lamb leg (without the bone)

4 sprigs thyme

1 tsp. dried rosemary

2 tbsps. mustard (whole grain)

1 tbsp. keto maple syrup

1/4 cup olive oil

1 tsp. garlic (minced)

Sea salt and freshly ground pepper to taste

Instructions:

1. Cut three 1-inch deep slits along the top of the lamb. Rub it with the maple syrup, mustard, salt and pepper. Make sure to evenly coat all sides. Then insert a combination of the garlic and rosemary into each slit.

2. Place the lamb in a crock-pot and cook on low for 7 hours. Then add the thyme and cook for another 1 hour.

3. Remove from the crock-pot and let it rest for 5 minutes before slicing.

Nutrition Information

Serves: 6

Calories: 414 (per serving)

Fats: 35g, Net Carbohydrates: 0.5g, Protein: 27g

Fish and Seafood Recipes

Keto Baked Herbed Salmon

Ingredients:

2 lbs. salmon fillet (cut into ½ lb. fillets)

½ cup mushrooms (chopped)

½ cup green onions (chopped)

4 oz. butter

½ tsp. rosemary

¼ tsp. thyme

¼ tsp. tarragon

½ cup tamari soy sauce

4 oz. sesame oil

½ tsp. basil

1 tsp. oregano leaves

½ tsp. ground ginger

1 tsp. minced garlic

Instructions:

1. Combine the sesame oil, tamari sauce and all the spices. Put the salmon fillets in a Ziploc plastic bag and pour in the marinade. Refrigerate for at least 1 hour. Make sure the skin side is up.

2. Preheat oven to 350°F. Line a baking pan with foil. Arrange the fillets in one layer. Drizzle the marinade over the fillets.

3. Place in oven and bake for 12 minutes.

4. Meanwhile, melt the butter in a skillet over low heat. Add in the mushrooms and green onions. Stir until they are fully coated.

5. Take out the salmon fillets and top each with the vegetable mixture. Put back in the oven and bake for another 10 minutes. Serve immediately.

Nutrition Information

Serves: 4

Calories: 353 (per serving)

Fats: 23g, Net Carbohydrates: 2g, Fiber: 1g, Protein: 32g

Cheesy Tuna and Avocado Balls

Ingredients:

10 oz. canned tuna (drained)

¼ cup parmesan cheese

1 medium avocado (cubed)

1/3 cup almond flour

¼ cup mayonnaise

½ cup coconut oil

¼ tsp. onion powder

½ tsp. garlic powder

Sea salt and freshly ground pepper to taste

Instructions:

1. In a large mixing bowl, combine tuna, parmesan cheese, mayonnaise and all the spices. Mix until all ingredients are well incorporated.

2. Gently fold in the avocado cubes into the mixture. Avoid mashing the avocado.

3. Divide the mixture into 12 balls and roll them over almond flour, coating them completely.

4. In a skillet, heat coconut oil over medium heat. Then add the tuna balls when the oil is hot enough. Fry until they are brown and become crisp. Make sure to fry all sides. Serve immediately.

Nutrition Information

Yields: 12 balls

Calories: 135 (per ball)

Fats: 12g, Net Carbohydrates: 0.8g, Fiber: 1.2g, Protein: 6g

Creamy Shrimp Scampi with Spinach

Ingredients:

40 raw shrimp (large)

4 handfuls of spinach

2 tbsps. heavy cream

6 cloves garlic (chopped)

½ onion (chopped)

1 tbsp. parmesan cheese

2 tbsps. olive oil

2 tbsps. butter

Sea salt to taste

Instructions:

1. Soak the shrimps in a bowl of water. Then peel off their shells and remove the heads.

2. Heat the olive oil in a skillet over medium-low heat. Add in the shrimp and cook for only 2 minutes. Then transfer on a plate and set aside.

3. On the same skillet, cook the onions until translucent. Then add the garlic and season with salt.

4. Stir in the heavy cream, parmesan and butter. Cook for 2 minutes until it thickens, then add the shrimp. Stir well and cook for another 3 minutes.

5. Transfer the shrimp with the sauce on a plate. Then cook the spinach using the same skillet. Don't overcook the spinach.

6. Transfer the spinach on another plate and top with the shrimp and creamy sauce. Serve immediately.

Nutrition Information

Serves: 4

Calories: 390 (per serving)

Fats: 24g, Net Carbohydrates: 3g, Protein: 36g

Keto Coconut Shrimp with Sweet Chili Dip

Ingredients:

1 lb. shrimp (peeled, deveined)

2 tbsps. coconut flour

1 cup coconut flakes (unsweetened)

2 large eggs (whites only)

(Sweet chili dip)

1 ½ tbsp. cider vinegar

½ cup apricot preserves (sugar free)

1 tbsp. lime juice

¼ tsp. red pepper flakes

1 red chili (diced)

Instructions:

1. In a small bowl, beat the egg whites using a hand mixer. Continue to beat until soft peaks form.

2. Put the coconut flakes in one bowl and the coconut flour in another bowl. Gather the three bowls together. Then dip each shrimp in the coconut flour, then the egg whites, and finally in the coconut flakes.

3. Lay them on a baking pan that is greased or lined with foil. Arrange them all in a single layer. Bake for 15 minutes in medium heat. Then flip them over and bake for another 3 minutes or until the coconut breading turns golden brown. Set aside to cool for a few minutes.

4. In a small bowl, combine all the ingredients for the dip and mix thoroughly. Then serve the shrimp with the dip on the side.

Nutrition Information

Coconut Shrimp

Serves: 3

Calories: 377, Fats: 20g, Net Carbohydrates: 4.3g, Fiber: 5.3g,

Protein: 36g

Sweet Chili Dip

Serves: 5

Calories: 20, Fats: 0, Net Carbohydrates: 2.2g, Fiber: 5g,

Protein: 0.2g

Keto Crockpot Clam Chowder

Ingredients:

1 ¾ lb. baby clams

2 cups clam juice

¼ cup chicken stock

1 ½ cup heavy cream

8 oz. cream cheese

2 tbsps. butter

4 cloves garlic (minced)

2 ribs celery (diced)

1 shallot (thinly sliced)

1 onion (chopped)

1 leek (trimmed and sliced)

1 tsp. dried thyme

1 tsp. garlic powder

Sea salt and cracked black pepper to taste

Instructions:

1. In your crockpot, pour in the chicken stock. Then add in butter, all the vegetables and season with salt and pepper. Cook on low for 1 hour.

2. Meanwhile, combine heavy cream, cream cheese, thyme and garlic powder. Mix well until the cheese softens and there are no more lumps of cheese.

3. Stir in the clam, clam juice and cream mixture into the crockpot. Then cook for 6 hours on low. Serve immediately while hot.

Nutrition Information

Serves: 12 (1 cup each)

Calories: 183 (per cup)

Fats: 19g, Net Carbohydrates: 3.75g, Protein: 9.3g

Desserts

Pumpkin Pie Spice Cookies

Ingredients:

½ cup pumpkin puree

1 tsp. pumpkin pie spice

1 ½ cup almond flour

1 large egg

¼ cup salted butter

½ tsp. baking powder

1 tsp. vanilla extract

1/4 cup erythritol plus extra 2 tsps. for the toppings

25 drops liquid stevia

Instructions:

1. Preheat oven to 350°F.

2. In a mixing bowl, combine almond flour, erythritol and baking powder. Mix until well incorporated.

3. In a smaller bowl, combine pumpkin puree, liquid stevia, vanilla and butter. Mix well. Then add this mixture and an egg into the flour mixture. Mix until all the dough is formed.

4. Divide and roll the dough into 15 small balls. Place them on a cookie sheet lined with parchment. Then press them flat using your palms.

5. Place baking sheet in the oven and bake for 12 minutes.

6. Meanwhile, combine the pumpkin spice and extra erythritol using a spice grinder. Then sprinkle this over the cookies once you take them out the oven. Let them cool before serving.

Nutrition Information

Serves: 15

Calories: 99 (per cookie)

Fats: 9g, Net Carbohydrates: 1.7g, Fiber: 1.5g, Protein: 3g

Keto Lime Cheesecake

Ingredients:

(Crust)

½ cup almond flour

1 large egg (yolk only)

¼ cup butter (solid)

½ cup macadamia nuts

¼ cup erythritol

(Lime filling)

2 key limes (juiced)

Zest of the 2 limes

2 large eggs

8 oz. cream cheese

¼ tsp. liquid stevia

¼ cup erythritol

¼ cup butter (solid)

Instructions:

1. Preheat oven to 350°F.

2. Grind the macadamia nuts using a food processor. Then add almond flour and ¼ cup of erythritol. Pulse until thoroughly combined.

3. Slice ¼ cup of butter into cubes and add it into the food processor together with the flour mixture. Pulse again. Then add the egg yolk and pulse until the dough is formed.

4. Knead the dough with your hands, then divide them evenly to fill 12 silicone cupcake molds. Fill only about 1/8 of each cupcake mold.

5. Place them in the oven and bake for 5 minutes. Take them out and set aside.

6. In a mixing bowl, combine another ¼ cup of butter and cream cheese. Once thoroughly combined, add 2 eggs and beat together.

7. Add in the erythritol and stevia, then mix again. Finally, add the juice and zest of 2 key

limes. Mix until all ingredients are well combined.

8. Pour the cream cheese mixture on top of the crusts. Make sure to leave out a little space at the top so they don't spill when they rise.

9. Place in the oven and bake for 30 minutes. Allow them to cool before putting in the refrigerator. Refrigerate overnight. You can add extra lime zest as toppings when you serve them.

Nutrition Information

Serves: 12

Calories: 226 (per cupcake)

Fats: 21g, Net Carbohydrates: 2g, Fiber: 1g, Protein: 4g

Dark Chocolate Mint Ice Cream

Ingredients:

1 cup heavy cream

1/4 bar dark chocolate (grated or crushed into small chunks)

Several drops peppermint extract

½ cup light cream

½ tsp. vanilla

15 drops liquid stevia

Instructions:

1. Place a metal bowl or ice cream bowl in the freezer for about 4 hours. Then put in all the ingredients, except for the chocolate chunks, and combine thoroughly. Put again in the freezer for about 5 minutes.

2. Use an ice cream mixer to achieve the right texture. You can add 2 to 3 drops of green food color if you like it to be green. Finally, add the chocolate chunks or shavings when

the ice cream maker has only 3 minutes left
of mixing.

3. Transfer in a sealed container and put in the
   freezer for a few hours until it hardens.

Nutrition Information

Serves: 4

Calories: 295 (per serving)

Fats: 31g, Net Carbohydrates: 3.5g, Protein: 1.2g

Pecan Coconut Ice Cream

Ingredients:

1.5 cup coconut milk (unsweetened)

¼ cup pecans (crushed)

5 tbsps. butter

¼ cup heavy cream

¼ tsp. xanthan gum

25 drops liquid stevia

Instructions:

1. Melt butter in a medium pan over low heat. Once it turns brown, add crushed pecans, stevia and heavy cream. Stir until well incorporated, then remove from heat.

2. Transfer the mixture into a medium mixing bowl, then add xanthan gum and coconut milk. Whisk all together until fully combined.

3. Place mixture in the fridge to cool. Then transfer it into your ice cream mixer to achieve the right consistency. Transfer to an

airtight container and put in the freezer until it hardens.

Nutrition Information

Serves: 3

Calories: 319 (per serving)

Fats: 35g, Net Carbohydrates: 1.3g, Fiber: 2g, Protein: 0.7g

Keto Strawberry Ice Cream

Ingredients:

3 large eggs (yolks only)

1 cup fresh strawberries (pureed)

1 cup heavy cream

½ tsp. vanilla extract

1/3 cup erythritol

1/8 tsp. xanthan gum

Instructions:

1. Combine heavy cream and erythritol in a pot over low heat. Don't allow to boil. Remove from heat once the erythritol dissolves.

2. Beat three egg yolks in a mixing bowl using an electric mixer. Then gradually add the heavy cream mixture while beating. Add in the vanilla extract and xanthan gum once you've poured in all the heavy cream mixture.

3. Put the bowl in the freezer to cool then use the ice cream mixer to achieve the right consistency. Put back in the freezer for about 1 to 2 hours.

4. Fold the strawberry puree into the chilled cream. Avoid overmixing. Then transfer in an airtight container and put back in the freezer for about 4 to 6 hours or until it hardens.

Nutrition Information

Serves: 6

Calories: 178 (per serving)

Fats: 17g, Net Carbohydrates: 2.8g, Fiber: 0.5g, Protein: 2.3g

Snacks

Fried Brussels Sprouts with Spicy Dip

Ingredients:

1 ½ lb. Brussels sprouts

1 tsp. lime juice

2 oz. mayonnaise

0.5 oz. hot sauce or sriracha

Coconut oil (enough to deep fry the Brussel sprouts)

Instructions:

1. Wash the Brussels sprouts under running water, then drain on paper towels. Then cut them into quarters.

2. Preheat the oil. Once hot, throw in the Brussels sprouts and fry for about 6 minutes or until golden brown.

3. While frying, combine sriracha and mayonnaise in a small bowl. Make sure they are well combined.

4. You could either serve the fried Brussels sprouts with the dip on the side or you could pour over the sauce and coat the Brussels sprouts evenly.

Nutrition Information

Serves: 1

Calories: 167

Fats: 11g, Net Carbohydrates: 16g, Fiber: 7g, Protein: 6g

Cheddar Cheese Chips

Ingredients:

1 ½ cup cheddar cheese

Your choice of seasoning (Mrs. Dash Table Blend, for example, or salt and pepper, or paprika and cumin)

3 tbsps. flaxseed meal (ground)

Instructions:

1. Preheat oven to 425°F.

2. Cut cheddar cheese into thin sticks. Then form 2 tablespoons of the sticks into small mounds and place them on a parchment-lined baking tray.

3. Sprinkle the flaxseed meal and the seasoning on top of each chip.

4. Put in the oven and bake for 10 minutes. Then remove from the oven and set aside for 2 minutes to let them cool and become crisp.

5. Remove excess grease by putting them on top of a paper towel. You can eat them as is or serve with a salsa dip on the side.

Nutrition Information

Yields: 12 chips

Calories: 54 (per chip)

Fats: 5.6g, Net Carbohydrates: 0.5g, Fiber: 0.5g, Protein: 3.9g

Keto Capresse Salad

Ingredients:

1 large fresh tomato

¼ cup fresh basil leaves (chopped)

6 oz. mozzarella cheese

3 tbsps. extra virgin olive oil

Sea salt and fresh cracked black pepper

Instructions:

1. To make the basil paste, use a food processor to combine basil leaves and olive oil.

2. Slice tomato into 6 ¼-inch slices. Cut the mozzarella into 6 1-ounce slices.

3. Assemble the pieces by putting the tomato at the bottom, followed by the mozzarella, and then topped with the basil paste. Season with salt and pepper to taste. You can add an extra drizzle of olive oil.

Nutrition Information

Serves: 2 (3 slices each)

Calories: 405 (per serving)

Fats: 36g, Net Carbohydrates: 3.5g, Fiber: 1.5g, Protein: 15g

Summer Smoothie

Ingredients:

¾ cup coconut milk (unsweetened)

2 tbsps. golden flaxseed meal

¼ tsp. blueberry extract

½ tsp. mango extract

¼ tsp. banana extract

¼ cup sour cream

20 drops liquid stevia

1 tbsp. MCT oil

7 ice cubes

Instructions:

1. Combine all ingredients in a blender. Wait for the flaxseed meal to soak in some liquid before pulsing.

2. Pulse until all ingredients are thoroughly incorporated and the consistency is thick. Transfer on a glass and serve.

Nutrition Information

Serves: 1

Calories: 352

Fats: 31g, Net Carbohydrates: 3g, Fiber: 5g, Protein: 5g

Energizing Avocado and Cocoa Smoothie

Ingredients:

½ medium avocado

1 cup almond milk (unsweetened)

1 tsp cocoa powder

1 cup spinach

1 tbsp. hemp seeds

1 tbsp. MCT oil

½ scoop protein powder of your choice

10 drops liquid stevia

7 ice cubes

Instructions:

1. Combine all ingredients in a blender and pulse until smooth. You can add extra cacao nibs for texture if you like. Pour on a glass and serve immediately.

Nutrition Information

Serves: 1

Calories: 391

Fats: 32g, Total Carbohydrates: 14g, Protein: 20g

Conclusion

Thank you again for purchasing this book!

I hope this book was able to help you understand what you need to know before and during a ketogenic diet. This book aims to give you a proper start on the diet. Eventually, you'll have to modify it according to your personal experiences while undertaking the diet. Keep in mind that people have unique bodies and may respond differently to certain foods and methods. Continue to research and add more to your knowledge, as further studies are still being made about the keto diet.

The next step is to learn the other aspects of a healthy lifestyle. Since a diet is only one of them. Incorporate the keto diet along with the right exercise, proper sleep and other practices a person must do to achieve a well-balanced and healthy life. Remember, the right mindset while undertaking any diet plan is focused on the health gains rather than the weight loss. Keep focusing on achieving a healthy lifestyle and your desired physique will follow.

Finally, if you enjoyed this book, then I'd like to ask you for a favor, would you be kind enough to leave a review for this book on Amazon? It'd be greatly appreciated!

Thank you and good all the best!

Preview Of 'Leptin Resistance Overcome: 17 Simple Steps To Fix Your Leptin Resistance, Beat Obesity, Get In Control of Your Weight and increase your Energy'

Learn how to finally master your LEPTIN RESISTANCE, which will help you BURN FAT and BUILD MUSCLE all at the same time using the powerful and effective proven methods in this book today!

LIMITED TIME BONUS INCLUDED! Receive a FREE book on the top 20 secrets to dieting success and keep the weight off forever, ABSOLUTELY FREE!

This book will help you see that your leptin resistance condition is not permanent. It CAN be overcome! Through careful action and persistent steps taken in the right direction, you CAN overcome your resistance to leptin. I am here to give you hope that you can still realize your dream of losing weight!

Let me ask you – are you tired of being overweight? Can you no longer stand obesity and all of the negative consequences that it brings? Have you already tried countless diets, exercise programs, and weight-loss programs in order to overcome it, but to little avail? And to crown it all, it has just been revealed to you that you are resistant to leptin – a hormone that causes a decrease in hunger at the end of a meal and helps to balance energy in the body.

Enter this book...

This book will teach you all that you need know on the subject and how to start combating it. Through the years, much information has been gathered and a wealth of research and information that has investigated numerous methods of getting it under control. Doctors and health authorities have been consulted and have tried and tested many of the solutions they prescribed. And so, in this book, you will be presented with that great wealth of well researched information and solutions.

This book discusses in detail several solutions and cures that have worked for many. You will be pleased to hear that most of the cures described are simple changes that you can apply to your daily routine – all of them natural, safe, and healthy! Leptin resistance can definitely be overcome through natural methods (I know, because it worked for me and countless others!) and this is the core message that this book aims to deliver.

So take action and embark upon this journey of discovery and revelation. There is so much this book wants to share with you. There are so many wonderful suggestions and practical tips that you can start applying immediately. And if you do so, you will start seeing a beautiful change in your condition!

Start reading now, and start applying the techniques today. You have nothing to lose but a whole lot of weight!

Here is a preview of what you will learn in this life changing book...

- What Leptin Actually Is
- How It Functions In Your Day
- What Leptin Resistance Is
- How To Beat The Resistance
- Do You Need To Supplement Leptin
- Symptoms Of Leptin Resistance
- Possible Causes Of Leptin Resistance
- And Much, Much More!

Have a look at what others are saying about this book:

Brilliant book! It was very easy to read and helped me understand the importance of overcoming leptin resistance. I found this book particularly helpful because it was packed full of practical tips that I can apply straight away. It gave me a clear plan of what to do and I can't wait to start! It increased my motivation and confidence that I can definitely lead a healthy lifestyle. I loved how the book understood health challenges, and gave hope and help for a brighter future. Uzma

Search the book using the information below and start your journey to a better you!

http://justreadme.com/

Bonus download:

Get 'Learn the top 20 secrets to dieting success and keep the weight off forever' 100% FREE!

- Top 20 secrets to dieting success
- Practical advice on weight loss
- Tips to help you succeed
- Why these secrets are effective and much more!

Get FREE access now! Just search this page

http://justreadme.com/weightloss-bonus-keto/

Thank You

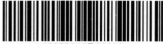

Printed in Poland
by Amazon Fulfillment
Poland Sp. z o.o., Wrocław